SEXY
FIT
&
FAB

at ANY age!

Praise for

SEXY, FIT & FAB at ANY age!

"Susie opens up new realms of possibility for women of any age to connect with their inner beauty and outer appeal. She introduces 8 simple and accessible keys to be the best you - living in your highest self at any age. Susie is a rare gem who walks her teachings and exemplifies what it means to be *Sexy, Fit and Fabulous at Any Age*."
~**Shajen Joy Aziz**, M.Ed., President of Transformational Inc., Author of Internationally Acclaimed book and documentary - *Discover The Gift*

"In this book Susie reminds us to be conscious about and realize how important it is as women to keep ourselves centered emotionally and fit physically, and from there we can exude our most confident, sexy, successful side. Feeling great about yourself from the inside out and the outside in breeds success in all facets of our lives."
~**Karla Keene**, CEO of ClarityRx Clinical Skin Care

"The real beauty of being a woman is that we have the innate ability to 'become' whatever we put our hearts to. *Sexy, Fit and Fab at Any Age* encourages true transformation from the inside out providing eight nuggets full of worthy essentials for every layer of life. "
~**Starla Faye**, Author, Publisher and *Two Talk Books* Radio Host

"Susie teaches you what it really means to be your best self, inside and out, and she makes it easy! I cannot think of a better person to write this book. Susie Augustin is the epitome of *Sexy, Fit and Fabulous!*
~**Ursula Mentjes**, Bestselling Author of *Selling with Intention*

"Susie Augustin encourages women to embrace their natural beauty and live a healthy lifestyle. *Sexy, Fit & Fab at Any Age* is about more than just looking sexy. When your mind, body and spirit are in harmony, you'll be radiant with self-confidence and others will be drawn to you."
~**John Maly**, Owner/President of Mirabella Beauty

"I thoroughly enjoyed reading *Sexy, Fit & Fab at Any Age* as Susie shares her 8 principles with honesty and expertise, which is relatable to every woman. This is a must-read as you will feel more empowered as you incorporate essential techniques and embrace your unique qualities!"
~**Nancy Ferrari**, Radio Personality, Life Coach

"Susie's book is filled with the tools and wisdom needed to fuel your confidence, embrace who you truly are inside and out and improve your life. She is warm, witty and reassuring. I highly recommend this book to women of all ages who want to feel inspired to move forward fearlessly while exuding beauty, confidence and sex appeal."
~**Kim Somers Egelsee**, Inspirational Speaker, Author of *Getting Your Life to a 10 Plus*

SEXY
FIT
&
FAB

at ANY age!

SAY YES TO YOUR
NATURAL BEAUTY
WHILE BEING FUNNY,
HEALTHY, SEXY & INSPIRED

SUSIE AUGUSTIN

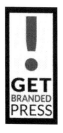

GET
BRANDED
PRESS

Get Branded Press
Long Beach, CA 90803
www.getbrandedpress.com

ISBN 978-0-9770018-1-1 paperback
ISBN 978-0-9770018-2-8 eBook
Library of Congress Cataloging-in-Publishing Data is available upon
request.

Printed in the United States of America
First Printing, 2013

Cover and Interior Design by Amy Pulliam (www.creativelinc.com)
Back Cover Photography by David Carlson

This book is dedicated to my mom
Betty Augustin
Thank you for introducing me to the
wonderful world of books and beauty, and
for always encouraging me to follow my dreams.

ACKNOWLEDGMENTS

I developed this book after speaking to a group of women about health, beauty and sex appeal. Kim Somers Egelsee, thank you for being an amazing inspiration, for your support and encouragement to live my life purpose, and for inviting me to speak at Willow Tree Women's Circle. To all the guest speakers and members of Willow Tree Women's Circle, thank you for your inspiration and friendship. To Power Women Package with Kim and Danielle Augustin, thank you for the strength of sisterhood. To Monarch Mastermind, I have deep appreciation for your ongoing support and collaboration.

Sincere gratitude goes to Amy Pulliam, graphic designer and fitness expert, for the sexy, sassy book cover design and for getting me into *sexy, fit and fab shape!*

To Amanda Russell, thank you for the thoughtful foreword you provided, you are a true inspiration to anyone wanting to look and feel their best, no matter what their obstacles or circumstances. Your *Hot Body Fitness* workouts are keeping me in amazing shape, thank you!

During the creation of this book, I met a several women who I admire for their vision and inspiration. My deepest gratitude to Shajen Joy Aziz for guiding me to not only discover my gifts, but to actualize them; to Ursula Mentjes for being intuitive in helping me prioritize my goals; to Starla Faye for your spirit and support of writers; to Tiffany Hendra for inspiring women to confidently move forward no matter what their story; to Hidi Lee for encouraging women to look and feel sexy; to Deborah Kagan for inspiring all women to live a sensual life; to Nancy Ferrari for supporting women in discovering their true essences; to Doris Muna for helping me get my mind, body and spirit in balance; and to Karla Keene for being my mentor in the beauty industry for several years and for helping me develop my full potential while becoming a Beauty Expert.

To my girls who embrace being *Sexy, Fit and Fab at Any Age,* thank you for your friendship, support and inspiration: Shaeny, Kim, Danielle, Taylor Doll, Shirley, Diane, Beth, Kristen, Natasha, Amy, Andrea and many more!

TABLE OF CONTENTS

FOREWORD

I'm inspired to write this after reading *Sexy, Fit & Fab at Any Age* because it elevated my mood, confidence and motivation for feeling fabulous. Being in the spotlight constantly, I love to stay fueled for success by reading books that encourage me to be myself, motivate me to feel beautiful, stay spiritual and indulge regularly in self care. Susie's book does just that.

In the chapters "Nutrition" and "Exercise", Susie shares personal stories of obstacles she overcame and choices she made to get physically fit, as well as tips to staying on track. I too understand the challenges women face in staying fit, as I had to overcome huge obstacles when I was considered in my prime fitness level. I suffered a career-ending leg injury as I was closing in on the Beijing Olympics for the 10,000m, and the doctors told me I would never run again. It was this fall from grace and the journey back where I realized fitness is about so much more than merely exercise. It is a catalyst for positive change in your life, and it fueled a new career for me, to share this with others via *The ARfit PRogram* and my weekly online YouTube show *Amanda Russell TV.*

I feel it is important that as women we uplift and support one another, and as a result, we feel great about ourselves. Paying someone a sincere compliment, working out with a friend regularly or hosting a spa party for girlfriends are all ways to amp up your confidence. Like Susie, I know the importance of treating your body, mind and spirit like royalty. Doing this helps you live by example and succeed in all areas of your life. The important thing is to realize that we all have beauty, we all have talents and we all have passions. We do not need to compare ourselves to others, but instead find our own and make the most of them. Susie's book teaches you just that. I do that in my work also. Think about ways you can elevate the world too, just by being you.

To your healthy mind and body,

Amanda Russell
TV Host, Celebrity Fitness Expert - *Hot Body Fitness,*
The ARfit PRogram and YouTube show *Amanda Russell TV*
www.amanda-russell.com
www.theARfitplan.com

INTRODUCTION

Susie Augustin is a Beauty Expert with over fifteen years experience in the health and beauty industry. She is an author, speaker, educator, publisher, columnist, marketing copywriter and branding specialist. She studied theatre, acting and improv for ten years and is very comfortable in front of an audience. Susie has been a featured speaker at numerous workshops, with topics such as skincare, health, beauty, sex appeal, confidence building, writing and publishing. Having worked at some of the world's most well-known and top rated beauty companies, she's motivated thousands of women to look and feel their best, to embrace their sex appeal and to live a healthy lifestyle. Susie shares her own stories and challenges to inspire women to develop their essences, exude confidence, embrace their true selves and feel extraordinary.

This book was written to help you uncover the eight keys to being *Sexy, Fit & Fab at Any Age!* It's intended to support you in exploring your inner beauty while watching your confidence increase. Anyone can have it all. Are you ready?

The first key is Spirit – exploring faith, gratitude, and inspiration.
The second key is Nutrition – enjoying whole foods, hydration, and support.
The third key is Exercise – getting physically fit, active, and being in nature.

The fourth key is Education – earn a degree, read books, and use your brain.

The fifth key is Passion – follow your passion or purpose, career, and hobbies.

The sixth key is Personality – embracing your uniqueness, having a positive attitude, and a sense of humor.

The seventh key is Grooming – personal appearance including skin, hair, makeup, clothes and fashion.

Next we'll explore Sex Appeal – confidence, inner beauty and balance; what is sex appeal and how to get more of it, and having passion for life.

Prepare yourself for transformation. Learn how to make the most of your assets and discover your beauty from the inside out. Imagine the life you can have when you follow your passion. When you are self-assured, have faith, feel strong, and are happy, you'll exude a natural spark which is very attractive and alluring. You'll become magnetic and draw others to you. What you radiate out you will get in return.

Now don't disillusion yourself and just jump ahead to the fun, sexy chapter. Anyone can follow tips on how to be sexy but they may come across as one-dimensional and not very interesting if they are missing the essences of the first seven chapters. As you'll learn, true sex appeal is having balance. Someone who may appear to be average looking but embraces several different qualities is much more appealing than someone who is gorgeous with a great body but missing some brain cells, or even a sense of humor. That pretty face may be nice to look at for about five minutes before the boredom sets in.

Keep in mind, balance is important to being *Sexy, Fit and Fabulous*. We've all been guilty at one time or another of putting extra emphasis on something, for example exercise, to the extreme that it consumes us and it's all we do or talk about. There are times when it's necessary if we had let that area in our life slide for awhile, and we need to get back on track. But loosen up a little and make sure you are doing it for the right reasons. Competing with someone else or looking for perfection can be disappointing, as most women will still feel like they need to "lose those last five pounds". Who hasn't thought at times that their tummy was a little soft or their butt too big? It's time to banish those thoughts as you strengthen your self-confidence while you become *Sexy, Fit & Fab at Any Age!*

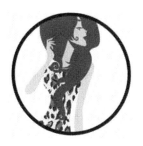

SPIRIT

SPIRIT

Spirituality is self-discovery, the inner path we take to get to know our true selves. Some enjoy meditation, yoga or visualization to get there. It's significant to be graceful and stay in faith- when your life is amazing, and even when you face hardships. Be open-minded to having a learning experience. It's possible that difficult situations are making you more resilient, getting you ready for your incredible life. Spiritual growth requires faith and gratitude, which can lead to you being an inspiration to others.

HAVE SOME FAITH

Faith is belief in and having trust in God, also known as the Creator, and being aware that there is more to life than what's going on in our own personal little world. Having faith can help get you through tough situations in life; you can get to the other side better and stronger. To strengthen my faith, I choose to listen to, watch, and read spiritual and inspirational CDs, DVDs and books. Others choose to join a church or a group of positive people who practice spirituality. Another suggestion is meditation and journaling, which will clear and quiet your mind of negativity.

Prayer can be powerful, especially when done on a daily basis. Some pray just when they are in predicaments, but be aware that prayers aren't always answered the way we want. It's not like rubbing the genie lantern and making a wish. Sometimes we focus on wanting others to change, or on situations that are out of our control, but it can be like spinning your wheels and getting nowhere. The key is how *you* can change and grow, becoming a stronger person.

AN ATTITUDE OF GRATITUDE

Gratitude is something that when practiced daily will become stronger and stronger, improving your life. When we appreciate the little things in life we feel happier and our troubles seem to be further away. When we obsess over our problems, we magnify them and they get bigger and

SEXY, FIT & FAB AT ANY AGE   5

worse. Be grateful for all your blessings, from good health to an income or having a family to love.

Living in an attitude of gratitude makes you feel more thankful, joyful and uplifted. You then in turn uplift those around you, as it's always more enjoyable to be around someone who is thankful than one who is feeling sorry for themself.

INSPIRE AND GET INSPIRED

When you are living a life of faith and gratitude a light shines from within you and you become a living example, an inspiration to others. When you have genuine compassion for others and you're as interested in what is happening in their lives as you are in your own life, people are drawn to you and want to know you better and have you in their lives.

Be thankful you can inspire others, as it's really a two-way street. You'll start attracting to you those who will be an inspiration to you, or become a role model, and they may help you on your path. I enjoy helping my friends with their writing, from editing their work, offering ideas or writing press releases for them. In turn, they or someone else will inspire me to make some positive changes in my life, or I may receive valuable suggestions that help me with my projects.

RENEW YOUR SPIRITUALITY

I renewed my spirituality a few years ago when I was feeling overwhelmed, overstressed, and it felt like there was nothing to be grateful for. I was feeling the aftereffects of divorce, experiencing financial struggles, had gone back to school full time, was dealing with challenges at work, and driving a salvaged vehicle. I thought I was making the best of things, struggling through, but I had a "survivor mentality".

My sister-in-law Danielle urged me to read an inspirational book that impacted her life, as the message encourages you to increase your faith and practice gratitude as you follow your dreams, and to not let the past or unexpected obstacles get in your way. I learned that you can change your life and you can make the choice to be happy.

I also started attending Kim Somers Egelsee's Willow Tree Women's Circle, a monthly workshop that helps women get their lives to a "10 Plus". It combines business networking with supporting other's journeys in a non-competitive environment. I learned that renewing my faith and practicing gratitude changed my life and the doors of opportunity opened up for me.

I was invited on numerous adventures and fun trips, including one to Maui just one week after I graduated. Fantasies of my upcoming trip got me through those last few months of school, and I now have a marketing degree that I'm using in amazing ways. I have a super positive circle of friends and business contacts, and I have a fabulous new car to get me around. I recently had an incredible night out at a charity gala with fun pictures and new friendships to show for it. I was also one of the contributing authors of *2013 Zoe Life Inspired: A Daily Devotional.*

SPIRIT TIPS

- Choose one positive new habit to do every day for a month; for example, write in your journal every morning.

- Make a list of 5 things you are grateful for.

- Help someone achieve their goals; for instance, I could write a press release for a friend with a new business.

- Let someone know that they've inspired you.

- When driving in traffic, listen to an inspirational CD instead of listening to music or talking on your cell phone.

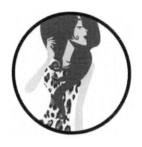

NUTRITION

NUTRITION

Nutrition is the food energy source we take in to make our bodies function. Some treat their bodies with kid gloves and others treat theirs without too much concern about the long term effects. We've all experienced busy schedules, stress and the convenience of the fast food drive-thru, and have not always been conscious of the nutritional value of what we are putting in our bodies.

Good nutrition consists of eating whole foods, staying hydrated and getting support if we need it. It's having the right balance of nutrients - carbohydrates, proteins, fats, vitamins, minerals, water and fiber, without excess of the wrong foods that can contribute to health problems.

EAT WHOLE FOODS

Eating whole foods is essential to receiving all the vitamins and minerals our bodies thrive on, and not just relying on multivitamins or supplements. We should be eating whole foods, grains, beans, vegetables and fruits. Some find that vegetarian or vegan lifestyles serve them well. If you want to eat animal foods, be sure they are high quality or organic.

To establish better eating habits, you can start adding healthy food to your diet, making you less hungry for the junk. You'll feel more energetic when you fuel your body with vegetables and grains, rather that grabbing that candy bar that tastes wonderful going down but leaves you feeling guilty, a little sleepy, and on the way to weight gain. Be sure to keep little snacks with you on busy days so that you don't forget to eat. Don't deprive yourself, or you may be more likely to binge and eat and drink junk food, sodas, sugary or fatty foods, and alcohol.

I'm known to take pleasure in a nice glass of wine. However, I'll consciously enjoy it on the weekend with a nice meal, not during the week in reaction to a stressful day at work. And, if possible, I'll make the choice to drink organic wine which is a great partner to organic dark chocolate. Just don't drink the whole bottle and eat the whole bar of chocolate, you may regret it in the next day. Did I say too much?

MAKE WATER YOUR FRIEND

Water is essential to staying hydrated and it helps your body function properly. It aids in getting rid of wastes through urination, bowel movements, and perspiration. It protects your spinal cord, lubricates your joints, regulates your temperature, and replenishes the fluids you lose from daily activities. Flush toxins out of your system by drinking plenty of water every day.

Drinking more than enough water will also show up in your skin. We hear about drinking at least eight cups of water a day, but that's just the minimum. I like to challenge myself to drinking 10-12 cups of water daily. I know, I know, people will look at you like you have a medical condition when you're running to the restroom every thirty minutes, but trust me, you'll look and feel great. A hydrated, healthy-looking and glowing skin is a side effect of a hydrated and healthy body.

HAVE A SUPPORT SYSTEM

Getting proper nutrition can be confusing as we are bombarded with advertisements for fast food and soft drinks. A lot the books out there written by experts have conflicting information. If we gain unwanted weight we're left even more confused, angry and frustrated. One day it's all protein with no carbs, the next week the fad is lots of carbs but low fat.

A nutritionist or a health conscious friend can teach you about the benefits of proper nutrition. Plus, they'll usually show you pictures of when they looked out of shape and awful, making you feel a tad better. Getting support and nutrition education will motivate you in your new healthy lifestyle. You can also educate yourself on nutrition by doing research online or reading books. Try out a new healthy meal plan and see how different you feel. It's also important to understand comfort food and what type of stress triggers emotional eating.

FROM FRUMPY TO FABULOUS

A few years ago I had weight issues of my own to deal with. I'd gone back to school to get my degree in marketing in an accelerated online program. For over two years I had a new class every month, homework every night, and spent my weekends writing essays and taking exams. There was no time for a social life and I was a little stressed out. At the same time, I made some career changes, leaving sales behind and diving into marketing. I was constantly being tempted by yummy comfort food at work – chocolate, candy and cookies. I quickly gained weight and looked and felt tired and frumpy.

About this time I found out my high school reunion was coming up shortly. I wanted to go, but not the way I looked or felt. I wanted my younger body back and I needed to lose thirty pounds.

I decided to ask for support from my friend, graphic designer and physical fitness expert, Amy Pulliam. We discussed my health goals, what I wanted to accomplish and why. She put me on a meal plan and workout routine. With determination I visualized daily what I wanted to look and feel like. Four months passed quickly and I accomplished the goals I'd set. I loved looking and feeling *sexy, fit and fabulous*, inside and out. At that point I didn't even care that much about my reunion, although I did go and totally rock the house, with my new fit body and fab hot dress! Don't be afraid to ask for help or support when you need it.

NUTRITION TIPS

- Buy organic fruits and vegetables this week.

- Challenge yourself to drink 8 glasses of water every day for one week.

- If you drink sodas, even diet, replace them with green tea.

- Ask one of your healthy friends what they do to keep in shape.

- Be a positive role model for others who want to eat healthier.

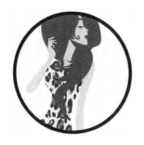

EXERCISE

EXERCISE

Exercise is necessary for your health and longevity. It's not just about getting skinny. Our bodies need exercise to function at an optimal level. It increases our stamina, keeps our muscles strong and toned, and can prevent health problems and diseases.

Who am I kidding? We all long to look amazing, fit and fabulous! Most women enjoy being a bit curvy, voluptuous and feminine. Looking and being fit makes you look years younger and feels good all over. Exercise also supports mental well-being since it increases your feel-good endorphins. It increases circulation in the body and the skin. Your skin will look radiant and glowing with that extra blood flow. Go out and have fun creating new habits being physically fit, active and in nature.

REPLACE FLAB WITH MUSCLE

To get or stay physically fit, you'll want to exercise at least 3-5 days a week. If you're super obsessive or have outrageous weight loss or fitness goals, you may be one of those who exercise daily, sometimes more.

The important thing is to just start. Creating momentum makes it easier to stay on track. Most women prefer cardio fitness to weight training, but be sure to add in strength training as it builds muscle, burns fat and speeds up the metabolism.   Who wants bye-bye arms? You know, on those bad days when you wave your arm and the flap of skin underneath won't stop waving? A great tip while toning your arms is to use self-tanner as it gives the illusion of better muscle definition and makes you appear slimmer.

I've always enjoyed exercise at home; videos, DVDs, I loved them all! Now with the advancement of technology you can get exercise on YouTube, not to mention the launch and trend of apps. They are the new DVD and getting even bigger - it's all about online shows and apps. My favorite app is *Hot Body Fitness with Amanda Russell,* it's great for home workout, on-the-go, and travel. These videos are fun and motivating; Amanda's variety of fitness methods are helping me stay in shape in less time than traditional exercise. We can all use more time, right? The benefits are getting toned and flattening the belly, increasing your metabolism, all while feeling and looking fabulous.

GET MOVING

Being active is a great way to start the morning or end the day feeling wonderful. Eliminate some of the TV watching, surfing the internet, and chatting on the phone. Have fun and take a dance class, be it salsa or swing, and you may even meet someone cute and interesting. Take up a sport like tennis, softball or swimming.

You'll find that adding activities to your lifestyle makes you feel more alive and is much more rewarding than a sedentary lifestyle. Enjoy yourself while you reach your ideal weight. One friend of mine likes to go to the golf range and hit golf balls, as it's technically exercise but also helps to release aggressions. I think she really goes to flirt, so hey, getting fit and a date at the same time is great for the ego.

NATURE GIRL

Being in nature can improve your mental health and self-esteem. From gardening to bike riding to fishing, being outdoors is enjoyable. Try hiking, it's great for the body and good for the mind. Go on a walk and take pleasure in all that nature has to offer. From enjoying flowers and trees, a lake or the ocean, nature takes you out of your head and it helps lesson anxiety. Walking at the beach is my personal favorite. I do it first thing in the morning and as I start out I'm usually thinking about the day ahead of me, or I may be thinking obsessive thoughts about work or the day before. The clean ocean air clears my mind, leaving me with a smile to start the day.

I also like roller skating at the beach. That's always a great conversation starter – guys think I'm out doing roller boogie wearing pink satin short-shorts with a tube top! They don't need to know that I'm actually wearing men's baggy sweat pants with an oversized t-shirt do they?

VISUALIZE YOUR NEW SEXY BODY

Think about what you want your body to look like and start visualizing. When I wanted to lose quite a bit of weight, I kept a picture of Jennifer Aniston nearby for motivation. In this picture she looks gorgeous, fit and strong. She has a reputation for eating healthy food and being devoted to exercise. In addition, she's talented, seems personable and has a great sense of humor, so who wouldn't want to be like her? When my resolve would start fading and I wanted to reach for a donut, I'd look at the picture of Jennifer to stay on track. While I didn't turn blonde, I did look like the best version of me. I'm not naturally lean, but a bit curvy. I learned to embrace my curves and enjoy my new fit body. Now, when I overindulge and want to melt away those extra pounds, I'll look at recent pictures of myself looking my sexiest for inspiration. Thanks Jen.

EXERCISE TIPS

- Work out every other day for 20 minutes for 2 weeks and see how empowered you feel.

- Start lifting light weights, even if you have to start with 3 or 5 pound dumbbells.

- Spend time in nature; go walking in the park, at the beach, or in the mountains.

- Find a fun exercise or dance on YouTube that will get your body moving.

- Visualize what you want to look like; you can collect pictures of fit and sexy celebrities that inspire you.

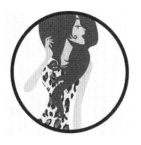

EDUCATION

EDUCATION

Education is significant in our lives. Learning activates the brain muscles and keeps our minds active. Studying and learning keeps us sharp, improves our decision making process, encourages independent and critical thinking.

Education can open up opportunities and can be pursued in several different ways. Make it fun and challenging. Your mind is like a secret weapon, no one else knows exactly what you've got hidden in there. You can obtain a certificate or degree, take classes or read books to expand your mind, all while staying young by using your brain.

EARN A CERTIFICATE OR DEGREE

It's never too late to go back to school and it's never too late to learn. Continuing your education gives you an amazing sense of accomplishment. Get a certificate, license or degree in something you are passionate about. Take online classes or go to the community college. You can take extension classes such as magazine writing or ceramics.

Your self-esteem will increase when you take on such a challenge. Continuing your education will open you up to new opportunities and a higher income. Unlock your potential and become the success you were meant to be. Make the investment in your future – there is no time like now. I earned my bachelor's degree while in my early forties and I'd never looked or felt better – knowledge is very sexy!

TAKE CLASSES OR READ BOOKS

Take classes in something you enjoy like finance, marketing or teaching. Your interests may be cooking, sewing, gardening, acting, or art; whatever it is, express yourself. If you don't like to read but love music, you can take up an instrument or join a band.

Whether striving for improvement or advancement, you can learn more about the field or industry you're in. You can also teach or educate others, which will give you a big sense of accomplishment. I love reading books on copywriting, marketing and self-publishing; it reinforces what I'm already good at and gives me that extra edge.

STAY YOUNG USING YOUR BRAIN

When you train your mind you can stay young by using your brain. I'm not suggesting you sign up for a calculus class. Reading, studying art or music is also training your mind. Know that knowledge is power. When my dad was in his mid-seventies he took a Photoshop class and learned how to use a laptop!

Challenge yourself and increase your intellect with learning. Take the first step toward a happier, more productive life. You'll gain self-confidence knowing you've become an expert.

HAVE THE GUTS TO GO FOR IT

Several years ago when I was facing divorce, debt, and disappointment, I realized that I had options in life. I attended Cal State Fullerton right out of high school and studied theatre for four years; acting, dancing and makeup, but I didn't graduate. Not having a degree kept me from moving forward in my career and I decided I didn't like feeling like a failure over my life choices and circumstances. A friend of mine went back to school in her forties to earn her bachelor's and master's degrees, and changed careers to become a teacher, proving to me that anyone can pursue education at any age.

I made the decision to go back to school and went for it. My goal was to get a marketing degree and to graduate with honors, all while working full time. Wow, the pressure we put on ourselves! It was my choice to focus on my career and studies, and I put my all into it. You can do this and have other things going on in your life too; just maybe less sleep or less time for friends and dating. This was a small sacrifice in the big picture.

I was thankful for my writing skills which helped me succeed both in school and at work. Once I graduated I was advised to set my sights higher and not to choose a career as a writer if I wanted to make any money. I'm glad I didn't listen because I make a living as a marketing copywriter, I write books and I inspire women through my speaking. I also teach workshops on how to write and publish books. There are times when we need to have the guts to follow our dreams even when some think we are being irresponsible.

EDUCATION TIPS

- Sign up for an online class; social media, how to market your business, etc.

- Find out if your job pays for continuing education.

- Read a book or buy a magazine about the industry you're in. I enjoy reading *SUCCESS* magazine, and it comes with a CD that I listen to in the car.

- Write an article about your specialty.

- Take a cooking class or go wine tasting; you can be educated on what wines go with what dishes.

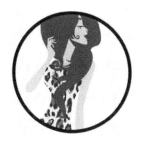

PASSION

PASSION

Living your passion will bring you remarkable results. Is your life rewarding, filled with passion or purpose? If not, what's holding you back? Sometimes the burden of responsibilities, bills, kids, or your job can make you feel stuck. You'll come to life when you follow your passion or purpose, enjoy your career and have hobbies that you take pleasure in.

PASSION OR PURPOSE

What do you feel passionate about? What do you love doing? Ask yourself some questions to figure it out if you're unsure. For instance, if you won the lottery, what would you do? I'm talking about after you bought a mansion and a sports car. Would you still work? Would you start a business, a non-profit, volunteer, help those in need, or write a book?

Answer these questions to feel clear on what your passions are. If I won the lottery, I'd start an art and writing non-profit program for kids, teaching them how to write and illustrate books. I'd also continue to empower and inspire women to follow their passions. Start taking steps to pursue your dreams. When you do what you love you'll have an inner glow, contentment, and you'll radiate confidence – it will draw others to you.

LOVE YOUR CAREER

Some people have been blessed with stability and are with their companies for decades. Others of us have reinvented ourselves a few times over and have experienced a few different careers. Are you in the field or industry that you want to be in or are you doing what was expected of you? If you had all the money you needed, would you continue what you're doing for a living? If not, what would you do?

You can choose to get even better at your job to get a promotion or advancement. When you become an expert at what you do your income and confidence will increase. Talk to others who are in the same line of work you're in or want to be in. Find out what obstacles they've overcome and what has made them successful. They may have suggestions about classes, books, or seminars that may help you.

ENJOY YOUR HOBBIES

What do you love to do? Do you enjoy graphic design, math, or gardening? Could you turn your hobby into a career? Go for it! When we enjoy our hobbies we're happier, more relaxed, and have a more satisfying life.

Years ago I dabbled in ceramics and got pretty good at my unique designs. I applied for a business license and sold my grape-themed coasters and serving trays to the wineries in Temecula. While I didn't make a profit, I did get a confidence boost in my artistic abilities. That led me into painting with acrylics on canvas and I focused on mermaids and beach themes. I started a new side business, Mermaid Studios. I gathered up my courage and I wrote, illustrated and self-published *Dolly the Mermaid,* a children's book for my niece, Taylor. It's one of my proudest accomplishments.

LIFE EXPERIENCES ARE LIKE PUZZLE PIECES

Life can sometimes be like a big jigsaw puzzle, all these pieces that don't seem to relate to each other or fit together. Throughout the years, I've had many interests and passions, and have done several different things. Now that I can connect the dots, or look at the whole picture, everything I've done has led to where I am now. I feel blessed that my passions, career and hobbies have intersected with each other and that I'm able to make a living doing what I enjoy.

When I was eleven years old my mom became an Avon Lady and introduced me to the world of skincare and makeup – I was obsessed. For several years I pursued acting and makeup artistry, and the confidence I gained on stage helped me tremendously in sales and education. My presentation skills prepared me to speak to and train thousands of women (and men) in the beauty industry, from product knowledge to sales training. I earned my aesthetician license and certification in permanent makeup, increasing my passion for skincare and the beauty industry. My makeup experience helped me to become a better artist, resulting in my illustrating and writing a children's book. Honing my writing skills came in handy when I went back to school to earn a marketing degree. Working for my dad in the printing industry made the transition into advertising and marketing very seamless. Being a marketing writer and consultant in the beauty industry was a no-brainer, as I'd become a Beauty Expert. Writing websites, brochures, ads, sales and education materials for beauty brands has made it a smooth conversion for writing for small businesses that need creative copy. This led to the development of the writing and publishing workshops I created, as well as the publishing company I started. I've also been speaking at numerous events including Mom Entrepreneur Success Conference, Willow Tree Women's Circle, and an upcoming Transformational Inc Event. I feel like I've come full circle with speaking, writing, publishing and sharing my message with women about being *Sexy, Fit & Fab at Any Age!*

PASSION TIPS

- Make a list of 5 things you'd like to do that you aren't currently doing.

- Write down what you would do with your life if money was no issue.

- What can you do to advance in your career?

- Can you make a living with your hobby, or have it become a part-time business?

- Make a list of your jobs and life experiences and see if they all make sense in the pieces of your life puzzle.

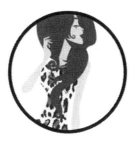

PERSONALITY

PERSONALITY

We all have our own distinctive personalities. From quiet to funny to serious to outgoing, the list goes on and on. A good personality is even more important than good looks because it reveals someone's true authentic self. People will want to be around you and work with you. It's important to experience the following to have a good personality: embracing your uniqueness, a positive attitude, and a sense of humor.

EMBRACE YOUR UNIQUENESS

Have the courage to embrace who you are. We are all different from each other with our own unique personalities. Some of us have our own style of dressing, ways of communicating, or an unusual laugh that sets us apart from others. If you're a dork, enjoy yourself and put your dork on a pedestal. Do not let teasing from others keep you from enjoying the quirks that are the essence of you.

I have a pretty loud and memorable laugh – I'd say that's what I'm known for. I own it and no one can take it away from me. I've had some light teasing, even some mocking over the years, and I'll admit my laughter got me kicked out of class more than once. Oh, I laughed all the way to the principal's office! It's interesting that when I see a friend I haven't seen for a very long time, the typical comment I'll get is, "I miss your laugh." This makes me happy that I stay true to myself. If you changed whatever that specialness is about you, you wouldn't be genuine. If everyone was the same in looks, personality and taste it would be a very boring world without the authenticity that brings the spice to life.

KEEP A POSITIVE ATTITUDE

Having a positive outlook will make you feel great. It takes less effort to focus on positive, empowering thoughts than it does to focus on negative, discouraging thoughts. Who would you rather spend time with; someone who is bitter and negative or someone who is happy, upbeat and makes the best of things?

Happiness is a choice, choose happiness. Find something to be happy about every day. I've been criticized for seeing the glass as half-full, for looking for something good in difficult situations. But that's okay, because I've had even more people thank me for helping or inspiring them. Smiling and being happy and positive pays off for everyone.

A SENSE OF HUMOR

Do you find humor in daily life? Do you laugh at yourself? Growing up I spent hours laughing with my best friend, Shaeny. Her mom informed us that only boring people get bored, so we found humor in everything and always kept each other entertained. We went to different schools, but we were both class clowns. It's hard not to be happy when you are always laughing and making other people laugh. We enjoyed physical comedy too, and had the bruises and scars to prove to what lengths we would go to entertain.

Practicing self-confidence, a sense of humor, and being positive will help you develop a great personality and others will want to be around you. A relaxed, happy and smiling face is easier to look at than a sour or sad face. If you're in a rut, you may need to fake it until you make it. Watch funny movies and experience how good you feel when you have a good laugh. Making others laugh makes them feel great, too.

PHYLLIS DILLER OR MARILYN MONROE?

The benefit of growing up in a large family of ten kids, and being an average-looking kid, is that I had to rely on my personality and sense of humor growing up. My heroes were Lucille Ball and Phyllis Diller. When I was eight years old my mom entered me in the Phyllis Diller look-a-like contest at Knott's Berry Farm, just so that we could get free tickets into the park. I wore a wild silvery gray wig and a sparkly silver dress – very Vegas-like!

I was also influenced by having seven brothers and learned things like burping and spitting. You had to become really good at these thing to show off and impress them, and I could burp louder than almost anyone. It paid off. While I did not get voted best looking or most popular in high school, I did get the *Pepto Bismol* award! I don't know if I should announce such a thing, but if I ever become a celebrity, some of the skeletons in my closet may be revealed anyway.

Now that I've painted that picture of myself, I'm sure you can imagine that it came as quite a surprise that as I was blossoming and coming into my own, men starting seeing me as sexy. I was a funny, burping, 18-year-old virgin, how could this be and what does sexy mean anyway? As I look back now I'd say that I must have been pretty confident in myself, who I was as a person, completely separate from my looks.

These days I'm more in touch with my feminine side, and am confident saying that I am not so average looking. I made the most of my looks, love how I feel and am told that I look gorgeous and sexy. I recently attended an amazing event with my friend Kim and we were asked to physically act out our childhood heroes without using words or sounds. Of course I was quite animated with my Phyllis Diller impressions. She was great, so funny and confident, always laughing. Kim thought I was being Marilyn Monroe, which goes to show that being funny and confident can be quite sexy!

PERSONALITY TIPS

- Write down what is unique about your personality.

- What kind of personality traits do you appreciate in others?

- Make a list of 5 positive things about you.

- Ask a friend what they feel are your unique personality traits.

- What type of sense of humor do you have - quiet, laugh out loud, dry wit?

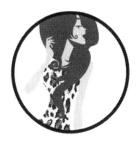

GROOMING

GROOMING

The value of grooming shows that you treat yourself well, and you know you are worthy. There's a time and place for being very natural and casual, and others times when making some effort is the better choice. Taking care of your appearance increases your self-esteem and it can improve the way others see you. It also makes it easier to look in a mirror. If you look like you have it together you come across as being confident; looking self-assured can open doors for you. Taking care of your skin, hair and makeup, clothing and fashion is basic grooming.

TAKE CARE OF YOUR SKIN

Start taking great care of your skin – prevention is key! The earlier in life you start the better, but it's never too late. Use the best products that work for you and protect your skin with SPF every day. Try mineral makeup for extra protection and a flawless look. Start using eye cream today, twice a day, it really does work. Do some research, not all effective products are expensive.

Drink lots of water and eat healthy food – it shows in your skin. I know, I know, we all hear of certain supermodels that chow down on cheeseburgers, drink endless amounts of diet coke and haven't exercised a day in their lives. Well, those girls are freaks of nature and who wants to look perfect anyway? I'm talking about the everyday, average woman. Us. We should take care of our skin because having clear, toned and moisturized skin will make you look younger. It will save you the money you were planning to use on Botox. You'll find that makeup looks even better and more natural on great looking skin, another reason to get on a good skincare regimen.

Some of us were forced into skincare and sun protection awareness at an early age. Growing up with auburn hair, freckles, and skin that sunburned, I felt like I was the first person in the 1980's to really embrace sunscreen. For years I was the only person I knew who used it consistently. Everyone made fun of me because I was the palest and it took me practically all summer to finally get a tan, but I didn't care. With my mom being an Avon Lady I had access to all the skincare products I wanted; cleansers, beauty masques, lotions, creams and sunscreen. In college, I trained all my friends to cleanse and moisturize their faces at night when we got home from parties and social gatherings. I'm so grateful I starting practicing prevention at an early age, as there is less for me to fix now.

HAIR & MAKEUP

Every so often save up and splurge on your hair. Do you know someone who always looks good? Find out who does their hair. Look at magazines, what do you like? What are you drawn to? Bring in pictures and be clear on what you like and don't like. Who wants their hair chopped off or all layered when they only have one thin layer to begin with? Have some fun with color or highlights.

Next, go to a cosmetics counter for a makeup lesson to find out what colors and looks are best on you, along with what you feel most comfortable with. When I was working in cosmetics and doing lots of events and makeup lessons, I found that most women like to feel naturally pretty every day, not look like a clown. Ask for makeup tips from your friends and find out what kind of eyeliner or mascara they wear, or what their favorite brands are. Know that you have a different, unique beauty.

MAKE FASHION FUN

Have fun with fashion without breaking the bank. There's nothing wrong with buying inexpensive clothes and these days there are more stores out there catering to those who are budget conscious. You can find clothes that are flattering by taking the time to try on various styles. Ask a trusted friend to go with you to find what looks best for your figure.

What does your look say about you? Are you conservative, fun, sexy, trendy, sporty, feminine or casual? Do you come across as being professional and confident? Does your look match what you're doing? If you're not into fashion, try to stay a little more conservative rather than wearing something wild and weird. Unless that's your style, then go for it.

Treat yourself to at least one great outfit – you're worth it! Keep in mind that fashion trends will usually cater to the young, their young bodies and shapes. What looks adorable on my 18-year-old niece will usually look awkward and unflattering on me, as well as make me look about ten pounds heavier.

WHAT'S YOUR STYLE?

My fashion sense is limited to a few signature looks. On dates, dinner with friends or even for business, I like wearing long dresses as they make me feel feminine and pretty.

They're flattering on me as well as comfortable (they call them maxi dresses these days, but don't these young girls know that I invented this look?) For meeting with clients, for work or networking, I like knee length black dresses that are professional looking, or if it's more casual, nice jeans, wedge heals and a black blazer. These are great looks that convey confidence. I've even seen my fashion forward friends copy this look. I have fun changing up my look with hair and makeup, I see them as accessories. A casual, cotton dress can be worn to the beach if you have on light makeup and a ponytail.

Spending time on making yourself attractive makes you feel good and attracts others to you. Usually we want our natural beauty to shine, but other times we want to look like a bombshell. Note that when you are sexy, some people can be put off or offended. It can be jealousy or insecurity, but sometimes it's because we've overdone it and too much sex appeal can be intimidating. For those who are naturally sexy and curvy, v-necks or something fitted can appear too much, even if it's not intended. It takes a lot of effort to look like a sex kitten and when it comes down to it, we really want to be liked for being our-selves, smart and funny, right?

GROOMING TIPS

- Use SPF every day on your face for a month; one meant for your face, not the kind you use all summer long on your body.

- Indulge in an eye cream; one that moisturizes, decreases puffiness and dark circles, or anti-aging.

- Give yourself a home facial, complete with a masque for your skin type.

- Have fun with fashion and buy a new sassy scarf.

- Go on a girl's night out and wear some sexy high heels.

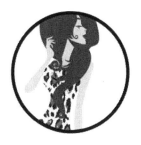

SEX APPEAL

SEX APPEAL

Having Sex Appeal is more than just being sexy, wearing a provocative outfit, or having a pretty face. When someone has the balance of mind, body and spirit they exude an inner confidence that is magnetic and very attractive. Sex appeal is also more than being attracted to another sexually. People want to be around others that are uniquely charismatic, with an inner beauty that radiates from them.

CONFIDENCE IS SEXY

Confidence is when you have self-esteem, feel self worth and accept yourself. People with self-confidence are typically optimistic, enthusiastic, assertive and independent. When we have a healthy self-image and believe that we have value, our self-esteem increases. Confidence does not mean that you think you are better than others, or even the best, but that you have belief in yourself.

People who are self-confident have the skill of inspiring or gaining trust in others. Self-confident people believe in themselves and do what they feel is right, even if others criticize or mock them. Setting and achieving goals is a great way to build self-confidence. I found my confidence increasing when I started spending more time on personal development and living my purpose. I was following my passions, learning what I needed to learn to further my career and surrounding myself with like-minded people. I created as much balance in my life as I could, living a healthy lifestyle, enjoying social activities and being happy.

INNER BEAUTY IS PRICELESS

Inner beauty is shown and expressed in many ways. Inner beauty is being kind and compassionate; it shows up in your smile and comes across as a sparkle in your eyes. While being attractive is great, it doesn't have very much value if what you have on the inside doesn't match what is on the outside. A pretty package is sometimes just that.

One can be very boring or one-dimensional if they don't have intellect and a pleasing personality. No one wants a shiny, red apple that is rotten on the inside.

Most women want to look and feel fantastic, their very best. I've always encouraged women to discover the natural beauty God has given them, to emphasize their strengths and to minimize, what they saw, as their flaws. I support women in embracing their inner beauty, as I believe that rejuvenation comes from the inside.

Last year I was asked to speak at Willow Tree Women's Circle about beauty and sex appeal. I instinctively knew I didn't want to focus on superficial beauty, so searched inside myself to find ways to communicate my message. I realized that I wanted to share my own journey, one through which I became confident, regained my looks and body, and felt empowered. I also wanted to encourage other women on their journeys to becoming *Sexy, Fit & Fab at Any Age!*

BALANCE – LIVE IN HARMONY

Creating balance in our lives can be bliss when we have it. Unfortunately, just like other goals or accomplishments we strive for, balance can go off-kilter when other responsibilities or projects come about. Also, when we become too consumed with certain areas of our lives, we somehow miss sight of other things that are important.

People will love you just for being who you are when you're embracing your natural beauty, letting your personality shine, along with those extra five pounds. We don't have to always obsessively diet, exercise and focus on our looks. Remember, at the beginning of this book we talked about the importance of balance, and a bit of moderation. By the way, what is it about women feeling they'd be just right if they lost those extra five or ten pounds? I look back at pictures of myself in college and think that I looked fantastic. Why did I believe at the time that I needed to lose five pounds? Now when I think I need to lose those extra five pounds, I smile with confidence knowing that I look fabulous!

Sex Appeal comes across when we balance the essences or keys we talked about in this book.

- Spirit – happiness and a positive outlook.
- Nutrition – eating well-balanced meals and drinking water.
- Exercise – getting physically fit and active.
- Education – pursuing knowledge or interests.
- Passion – enjoy your life, from your career to your hobbies.
- Personality – be confident in your true self and have a sense of humor.
- Grooming – take care of and have pride in the way you look.
- Sex Appeal – reveal your inner beauty, be confident and passionate about life.

Someone who has all this going on is bound to be sexy, alluring and self-assured! When I got my essences in balance my life started to really change and people saw my inner glow. I kept my sense of humor and pursued my passions. I started naturally oozing sex appeal and didn't realize it until women started asking me for tips on how to look and feel sexy. I was caught off guard, as I still see myself as the funny little girl dressed up like Phyllis Diller trying to get a laugh.

WHAT IS SEX APPEAL AND HOW TO GET MORE OF IT

In exploring what makes someone sexy, I took a look at celebrities and sex symbols, and came across some commonalities. One of the common traits of people who are naturally sexy is confidence in themselves; their looks, abilities, personality and talent. They are comfortable in their bodies and have a healthy self-image. Celebrities with sex appeal know how to move. They may have experience in theatre, dance, singing or performing. They have had years of experience and know how to turn it on. They come across as being confident, happy, with a good sense of humor. Having passion for life is very sexy!

Try some of the following tips to build your self-confidence and amplify your sex appeal.

TIPS TO BUILD YOUR SELF-CONFIDENCE

- Take a public speaking class.

- Change or improve your look.

- Visualize how you want to come across to others.

- Face your fears and have the courage to take a chance.

- Put the sizzle back in your passion.

- Pretend you are already confident.

SEX APPEAL TIPS
HOW TO BE SEXY, FEEL SEXY

🍸 Take a dance class; salsa, jazz, ballroom.

🍸 Get in touch with your body; take bubble baths with soft music, champagne and candles.

🍸 Wear sexy lingerie under your business suit.

🍸 Get a spray tan, it shows off your new muscles and makes you look skinnier.

🍸 Wear sexy high heels, your legs will look fantastic and they'll give your walk a wiggle.

🍸 Have the confidence to laugh out loud.

🍸 Give the aura of mysteriousness or inner sass.

🍸 Explore your inner beauty and watch your confidence increase.

Imagine the life you can have when you are
Sexy, Fit and Fabulous!

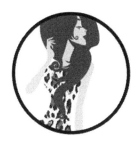

ANSWERS TO EVERYDAY QUESTIONS ABOUT
BEAUTY, CONFIDENCE AND SEX APPEAL

WHAT ARE WAYS INNER BEAUTY RADIATES OUT TO OTHERS?

How can that benefit us and them?

This is one of the questions that I'm often asked by women. First, let's address inner beauty. Inner beauty is the essence of us, what we have on the inside, our kindness, how we treat others, our unique qualities. Some believe that inner beauty is used to describe someone who is unattractive, but that's just nonsense. I understand that the subject of beauty can be very confusing in this day and age, as a lot of emphasis is put on outer beauty.

Someone who has inner beauty is kind and compassionate toward others and themselves. I'll repeat, inner beauty is being kind to yourself. As you take care of your inner self, your spirit, you'll begin to take care of all aspects of yourself.

When you believe in your inner beauty you will be radiating out to others your happiness, joy and compassion. When you are genuinely interested in another's unique essences, you form connections. What this does for others is validate them and in return they take a deeper interest in you. What I find is that when I have this type of true connection with others, I'm enthusiastic about helping them with their interests, and when I show my true self, others are right there to lend a hand, helping me in my pursuit of my passions. We end up helping each other to succeed.

WHAT ARE SOME SECRETS TO STAYING YOUNG, INSIDE AND OUT?

There are different ways to staying young. When you take care of yourself physically, with exercise as well as what you put inside your body, you will have more energy, feel lighter and be happy. What you put on your skin as far as skincare and makeup can help you continue to look young (or older, if you are using the wrong products). Add on top of that clothes that are flattering on you, and you'll have yourself a nice, healthy looking package.

But don't stop there. You need to consider your inner life, your spirit; take time to meditate, pray or journal. Fill your mind and thoughts with positivity. You'll also want to fill your mind with knowledge. Keeping your mind active with learning new things, reading books and taking on challenges; all will keep you sharp and feeling younger.

Following your dreams and accomplishing your goals will make you feel happy, vibrant and enthusiastic. You will be joyful and glowing, grinning from ear to ear, with a youthful like exuberance.

In addition to feeling young by the way you treat your mind and body, think about what you liked doing when you were a kid. Did you enjoy sports, singing, crossword puzzles or painting? Treat yourself to a day of doing some of the activities you took pleasure in as a child.

One of the things I loved doing as a kid was art projects; drawing and painting. I have several nieces and nephews, as well as friends with kids. The way I bonded with them was to sit on the floor with coloring books, or bring over some art paper and paints, or even do some mosaic projects. The kids loved it because they had my undivided attention as I encouraged them to have confidence in their creativity. I loved it because I felt like a kid again. Interestingly enough, all these kids associate me with being fun. Even years later when they've grown up, they remember the art projects I used to do with them.

A few years ago when I went back to school to get a marketing degree, my nephew Luke, who was about six at the time, asked me a very profound question. "Sisi, what are you going to be when you grow up? Would you say that you're an artist?" It was a very sweet and funny moment. We still enjoy doing projects together when I come over, and I've got to say, Luke is quite the artist as well as writer, and he has a collection of pig stories and drawings.

Earlier in the book I posed the question, "What would you do if you won the lottery?" I said I'd start a non-profit company for kids, with writing and illustrating workshops, teaching them how to write and publish a book. How about if I just go for it now? Help Luke create his book and publish it. I feel like I've come full circle, encouraging and helping out kids who love to do exactly what I loved to do as a kid. Saying I'm going to do something and going for that goal is one of my secrets to staying young!

HOW DO WE STOP COMPARING OURSELVES TO OTHERS?

Are we influenced by the magazines and TV around us? Media can sometimes be tough on us. We are bombarded with magazine and radio ads as well as TV commercials touting the latest diet pills, plastic surgery procedures and endless images of The Beautiful. We've been programmed to have an opinion on what is and isn't beautiful, the ideal body type and how we should look. It can be very confusing and damaging. When we see someone average looking on a TV show or magazine ad, we tend to be a little judgmental, thinking, "She's not that pretty."

Growing up I never felt like the prettiest, or even close. I had strange colored hair; lots of auburn, some brown, lots of blonde highlights from spending so much time outside, and it was a little curly and frizzy. I had freckles and skin that burned and took a long time to tan. But back then we didn't focus so much on our looks; we were busy playing outside, doing art projects, using our imagination. I enjoyed myself and loved having a good laugh. I had personality and confidence. In time my outer beauty grew stronger, matching my inner beauty. I embraced my unique look and my curves and my confidence increased.

We need to get to the place where we enjoy our uniqueness. I accentuate what I have going for me – my red hair will be the reddest, my curves will be rocking and you'll always catch me with a smile on my face, and most likely laughing!

DID YOU EVER GO THROUGH A FRUMPY PHASE?

How did you learn to be fabulous instead?

Throughout the years I've gone through a few frumpy phases. I think most of us go through different phases where we focus on certain parts of our lives; career, health, looks, love interest, hobbies, spirituality or family. It can be a challenge to find balance in our lives, many times something important slides, getting less attention than it should.

There are several different life experiences that can cause frumpy phases.

- Being comfortable in a relationship.
- Working a casual job that doesn't require you to look your best.
- Gaining weight and not feeling confident in your size.
- Overindulging during the holidays.
- Being in an unhappy marriage.
- Health issues.
- Being a mom.
- Letting your job consume you.
- Going through a divorce.
- Surrounding yourself with others who aren't concerned about appearances.
- Overwhelm and exhaustion.
- Being a full-time student.

I've experienced a few of these life experiences. During some of them I've gained a lot of weight but didn't look frumpy. I actually looked very put together, professional and polished. During other times, my weight was fine but my looks weren't my priority. Health issues were annoying because exercise was limited, and while in physical pain, wearing comfortable sweats was the best I could do. Sometimes when there are several exciting things going on in my life, my focus is on my passions and opportunities. I'm so busy with my creativity that I don't take the time with my appearance and I may go days without wearing makeup.

Don't get me wrong, I do care about physical appearance but it's not my priority. Having confidence in myself and knowing that I can look good when I need to, helps me rationalize looking frumpy. When I'm out running errands I'm on a mission and I don't take the time to get dolled up (or to sometimes even look half-way decent). I know that this is a choice I'm making at the time, so I'm fine with it and I give no apologies. That is until I unexpectedly run into someone that looks amazing, fit and beautiful and I kick myself for not wearing makeup or for wearing really comfortable (ugly) shoes. I usually just find humor in the situation. Recently I ran into my friend/hairdresser Robert in the supermarket. We had a quick chat and then he excused himself. When I caught sight of myself in one of the glass doors I started laughing – what a mess! I don't think he wanted to take any credit for my beauty (inner or outer) that day! Luckily the next time I saw him I looked like a bombshell. Remember, it's all about balance.

There are several ways to look and feel fabulous.

- First, you need to decide that's what you want.
- Start exercising to look and feel better.
- Get a workout partner.
- Buy some great anti-aging skincare products.
- Ask a friend to help or encourage you.
- Buy some new clothes that flatter your figure.
- Get a makeover.
- After your makeover, go home, raid your closet and play dress up.
- Wear sexy lingerie under your clothes.
- Put on some sassy hoop earrings.
- Flirt with someone you find attractive.
- Wear sexy high heels.
- Put on a dress that makes you feel feminine.
- Wear red lipstick.
- If you always wear black, wear color.
- Take the time and do it.

WHY IS BEING FIT AND HEALTHY SO IMPORTANT FOR YOUR SUCCESS, CONFIDENCE AND BALANCED LIFE?

Being fit and healthy is about so much more than having a sexy body. It's about balance, strength and longevity. With all of the preservatives, antibiotics, pesticides and hormones that can be found in our food these days, it makes sense to start making healthier choices. Poor nutrition is going to affect your health, mind and body, as well as your mood.

When you achieve success you want to be in great shape while you're reaping the rewards. Sometimes being in shape first is required, as being fit and healthy requires focus, discipline and creates strength. These are necessary attributes of a successful person.

To have a balanced life, there are many things you need to juggle. Your health, self-care, work, family, and spirituality just to name a few. If you neglect your health and fitness level a few different things happen. You're not setting a good example for those around you. By default of not getting the benefits of exercise, you won't look and feel as good. If all your time is consumed in other places, you may experience burn out.

What does being fit and healthy do for you? It gives you strength. Physical strength and mental strength. You never know what kind of curveballs life is going to throw at you. Personal, financial, losses, health issues. Difficulties are a lot easier to handle when you are mentally and physically strong.

Sometimes what's completely unexpected, even when you feel like you are in your prime fitness level, is health problems. Several of my friends and I have experienced this. What a frustration it is to get bad news from a doctor when you know you've been eating healthy and working out every day. After you do some research and are past the "why me?" phase, believe me, you will be very grateful that you are already in great shape and are able to handle things better. Nothing is scarier than having surgery, facing the unexpected, having your body repaired, or even having internal organs taken out. Recovery can be what you make of it. Will you feel sorry for yourself? Or will you be thankful that you have a strong healthy body that will recover faster than if you'd been neglecting it? Having a healthy lifestyle will help in your recovery as you will already have healthy eating habits that will carry you through, and keep you from making excuses to eat unhealthy comfort food. You'll bounce back quicker and find a life lesson in what you've experienced, maybe even talk to and help others who are going through something similar.

One of my favorite things about being fit and healthy is that you can be a great influence on others, inspiring them to make better choices. The nice thing is that when you go through weaknesses or temptations, they will return the favor and help lift you up.

WHAT ARE YOUR SECRETS TO CONFIDENCE?

Practice being bold, confident and self-assured.

Confidence can take on many forms but it's important to know who you are, what your values are, and being self-assured. I believe it starts with having a strong inner life, practicing spirituality and gratitude. If you don't already know what your talents and strengths are, ask a friend, teacher, family member or co-worker to help you out. What are you passionate about, what makes you forget about time and go into the zone when you do it?

Once you have a clear picture of who you are, feel proud of yourself for your talents and accomplishments. If you're just starting out and haven't done much to speak of, donate your talents and services. This can be to a friend, family member or the community. Giving makes both the giver and receiver feel great. The more you give of your talents, the more experience you gain, and the more your confidence increases.

As your confidence in yourself, your talents and beliefs increase, you will feel more bold and daring. Your imagination may run wild and you'll start seeing yourself accomplishing more than you'd ever hoped. You'll want to feel good, look good and take care of yourself. You'll start seeing yourself as this amazing package with great qualities and assets. If you haven't already, this is an ideal time to start setting some goals.

I love big lofty goals. But I also believe you need to map it out a bit. Set short term and long term goals. Tell someone you trust about your goals; this can help keep you on track and more inclined to take action.

When I'm creating my goals, I like to visualize what it will look like when I get there.

- How will I feel?
- Who will I be sharing this moment with?
- Where am I?
- What am I wearing?

As I see a clear picture, more thoughts come into my head. If my visualization shows me looking amazing, what step can I take to look that way? Work out more, start jogging, and eating better? I like to hold onto these feelings. Feel the happiness, joy, accomplishment and CONFIDENCE!

You can take these feelings with you anywhere! Dress for the part you want to play. Act "as if". As if you are already there, enjoying your life. Act confident and be confident.

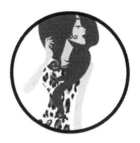

WHAT IS YOUR PLAN FOR BEING
SEXY, FIT & FAB?

TAKE STEPS TO BEING
SEXY, FIT & FAB

Below is a review of what was shared in this book. Now let's make a plan of action. What steps will you take to be *Sexy, Fit & Fab at Any Age*? Take some time to visualize what it will look and feel like. Write it down. Next, visualize the steps you will need to take to get there. Write down the steps, you can even doodle little drawings. Remember, stay true to yourself and have FUN!

Sex Appeal comes across when we balance the essences or keys we talked about in this book.

- Spirit – happiness and a positive outlook.
- Nutrition – eating well-balanced meals and drinking water.
- Exercise – getting physically fit and active.
- Education – pursuing knowledge or interests.
- Passion – enjoy your life, from your career to your hobbies.
- Personality – be confident in your true self and have a sense of humor.
- Grooming – take care of and have pride in the way you look.
- Sex Appeal – reveal your inner beauty, be confident and passionate about life.

SEXY, FIT & FAB PLAN

_____

_____

_____

_____

_____

_____

_____

_____

_____

_____

_____

_____

_____

_____

_____

_____

_____

_____

_____

_____

_____

_____

_____

SEXY, FIT & FAB PLAN

_____

_____

_____

_____

_____

_____

_____

_____

_____

_____

_____

_____

_____

_____

_____

_____

_____

_____

_____

_____

_____

SEXY, FIT & FAB PLAN

_____

_____

_____

_____

_____

_____

_____

_____

_____

_____

_____

_____

_____

_____

_____

_____

_____

_____

_____

_____

_____

SEXY, FIT & FAB PLAN

_____

_____

_____

_____

_____

_____

_____

_____

_____

_____

_____

_____

_____

_____

_____

_____

_____

_____

_____

_____

54517319R00061

Made in the USA
San Bernardino, CA
20 October 2017